SHIBARI FOR BEGINNERS

The Step-By-Step Guide to Mastering the Art of Kinbaku and Japanese Rope Bondage – Complete with Pictures of Every Step of Every Knot and Rope Play

Takeshi Shiba

Table of Contents

CHAPTER 1

Introduction: History of Kinbaku

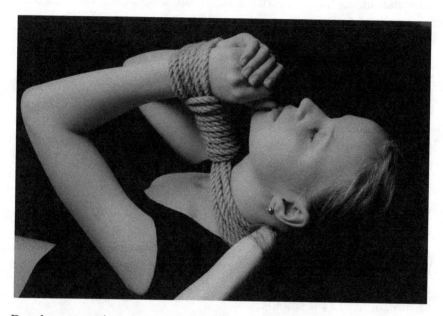

Bondage continues to stimulate many prejudices to this day. Sometimes it is associated with sexual practices and other times with torture and sadomasochism. While it can often come together, it does not always. Bondage has a long history of pleasure and art before becoming a defining component of modern BDSM.

Shibari, also known as Kinbaku, has its origins in Japan where the practice of the rope begins with Hojōjutsu. It is a martial art involving rope that was used by a class of samurai to capture and transport prisoners of war from the Edo period which took place between 1603 and 1868. In Japan, it is culturally natural to tie up since iron was a rather scarce resource. In this way, it was not possible to make metal handcuffs to hold the prisoners. The immobilization techniques were therefore used from the rope. However, the techniques used at the time are a far cry from what we can see today in more erotic contexts. They were mainly based on torture. It could even be used in death sentences where prisoners were immobilized in an awkward position that could torture them for hours, if not days, before they succumbed.

Many schools of Hojōjutsu have sprung up and each one practiced its own style. The patterns and techniques for tying gave a lot of information, such as the jurisdiction of the school, the social rank of the prisoner as well as the crime that was committed. This way, during public punishments, the crowd could know what it was about.

In the early 20th century, pain began to be adopted from an erotic point of view in Japanese theaters. It was not associated with what might be called sadomasochism, since the culture of the time put more emphasis on beauty and aesthetics. During these performances, the actors reproduced the Hojōjutsu in a safer and more aesthetic way to provide a memorable experience for the audience.

It was not until after World War II that bondage took on an erotic form, making its mark in erotic magazines. This new fashion made its introduction in the West around this period. This fetish will become more and more popular from that point on, both in Japan and in the West thanks to the unusual side of eroticism through torture, at least as it sounds.

In America, a different style, the western bondage, was created to suit a culture that mainly seeks to achieve a specific goal. The techniques in action are meant to restrict quickly and safely. The Japanese style, Shibari, focuses much more on the art and the flow of a session where the sensuality is much more present.

What can this book teach you?

This guide aims to introduce you to the art of Japanese bondage. It is primarily intended for a beginner audience who wants to learn the basics and precautions so that they can exercise in confidence and safety.

It is your responsibility to always use good judgment when doing bondage. The risks and possibilities of making mistakes are numerous. Just reading this book does not make you an expert and nothing can replace the training and feedback that comes from a face-to-face interactive course. You should know that tying comes with risk and that it is impossible to create a situation without the presence of danger. Make sure you are comfortable with the level you are starting out. If a dangerous situation arises when you are unable to react properly, there can be real consequences.

Language and terms used

Several terms are used in the field of bondage. When starting out in the industry, it is possible not to know them exactly and not necessarily be comfortable with them.

Practice:

Shibari - means "to tie" in Japanese

Kinbaku - means the action of tying up tight in Japanese

Semenawa - Japanese expression for rope torture, seme is torture and Nawa is rope in Japanese

The roles:

Top / Rope top / Rigger / Nawashi: Represents the person who ties or practices the art of tying.

Bottom / Rope bunny / Model: Represents the person being tied up

Switch: Represents the person who performs the action of tying as well as being tethered. They can reverse the roles at will.

The rope:

Bight: The middle of the rope which is obtained by folding the rope back on itself. It is usually from this point that we start

Rope end: The end of the ropes

Button: End knot so that the cords do not fray

Strand of rope: One half of the rope, when is fold and doubled, it is called a wrap

Rope flow: The part of the rope that is not yet used, between the bight and the rope end.

CHAPTER 2

All about ropes

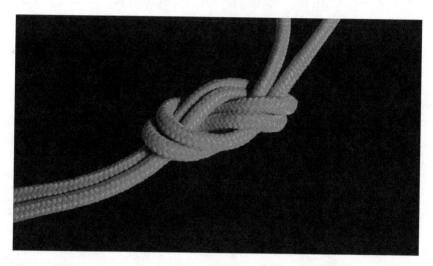

There are several types of ropes for different uses. Each has advantages and disadvantages that may not always be suitable for all situations. This part is about differentiating between each one and allowing you to find out which one is best for you.

Some strings will have greater stiffness and will keep their shape, even when there is great tension.

Conversely, some strings have greater elasticity and will stretch and thin under tension.

An elastic rope is especially to be avoided when looking for suspension. This is because it can stretch under the weight of the person posing a danger. During a suspension, a person's weight rests on the ropes. If the cords become thinner, the contact area is reduced and can cause pain. A stiff rope is much more predictable when tension comes into play and that is why it is used when there is high tension involved.

Plastic fiber ropes are strong and can withstand heavy loads but are not as soft on the skin as natural fiber ropes. They can therefore cause certain irritations on the skin. In addition, they cause burns more quickly on rapid movement (This part will be explained later).

Natural fiber ropes, although less durable, are generally more pleasant to the touch than plastic ropes. Also, be sure to take strings that do not contain any industrial oil. These can be irritating to the skin.

Most plastic ropes are inexpensive. However, the quality is low and is often limited to initiation and finding out if you want to practice deeper in bondage. If you are planning to experiment more regularly, you or your partner will want to switch to higher quality natural ropes.

The softness of a rope is a rather personal factor. For erotic and sensual games, soft ropes are more preferred. For games with a sadomasochistic tendency, rough strings can make you happy. Without going to one extreme or the other, some strings sit in the middle of the two to provide good feel while still maintaining a pleasant feel to the touch.

Another important point to keep in mind is how much friction you want your rope to have. Softer ropes will have less friction and will require tighter, more complex knots to hold. Rougher ropes will not need complex knots since they have a high friction factor.

Jute:

Jute rope is one of the most popular and is traditionally used for bondage. It is also one of the most accessible and easy to find among natural strings. It is medium soft and will not stretch under stress.

Hemp:

Hemp is another of the most popular in the world of Shibari. It is stronger than jute and softer. Usually, however, you will have a little more difficulty finding them. It should be avoided to encounter water, otherwise it could degrade quickly.

Cotton:

They can be found very easily and in many places. If in doubt, the nearest sex shop probably has some in stock. It can be useful in many situations because of its softness but has elastic properties. It is also an easy to clean rope since water does not degrade it in any way. It then becomes possible even to do bondage involving water.

Bamboo:

Among the softest ropes available, bamboo is also among the most expensive and difficult to obtain ropes. It is an elastic natural fiber that is not suitable for every session, but mainly for sensualism.

Sisal and Manila:

These ropes can be found in hardware stores but will likely have oils that are irritating to the skin. If you can manage to process them to make them more conformal, you will end up with rough and stiff ropes.

Coconut:

Arguably the roughest rope that can be found. It is ideal for people with a strong interest in sadomasochism. You will probably need to handle them with gloves, so you do not hurt yourself when you tie up.

Nylon:

In the bondage world, this is arguably the most popular synthetic fiber rope. It is soft, but also elastic. It can be compared to cotton on many criteria but stands out for its much higher resistance.

Polyester and Polypropylene:

Both types of plastic fiber ropes are quite easy to obtain, especially at hardware stores. They are inexpensive and can be interesting to start. They are very inexpensive, soft, but also elastic.

Hempex:

It looks like hemp and has the same texture but is made of plastic. It therefore allows greater resistance, but remains soft and, unlike most synthetic ropes, is rigid. On the other hand, to be able to get it, you will have to spend more.

- Rope length

The length of the rope will be important in the type of session you want to set up. The longer a string, the less connections you will need to make to extend the original string. However, you will reduce the speed for tying as it will be necessary to pull a large amount of rope with each step.

There are all kinds of ready-made lengths that are found frequently, like 4M or 8M. It is always possible to personalize them by cutting to the desired length. It is up to you to find the right length for the style you want.

- Rope width

Usually, the larger a rope diameter, the harder it will be to bend it over itself, tie knots and manipulate it.

Conversely, a thinner rope will offer little contact on the skin and cause pain more easily.

The most common ropes have a diameter of 5.5mm or 6mm. They are malleable and suitable for most situations.

Going towards a larger diameter is often an attempt to tie up a person who is more overweight and who might experience pain with a thinner rope.

Finally, 4mm ropes can allow more precise work and are not recommended for suspension since great tension can inflict enormous pressure on the skin.

Chapter 3

Types of recovery

To preserve a string and make it last longer, treatment is usually done for the strings. Plastic fiber ropes do not need it, while natural fiber ropes do. Otherwise, your rope may end up rotting. Like treated lumber, it lasts longer, so you do not have to constantly buy or re-buy material if you build it yourself.

There are several types of treatment, whether with oils or wax. Although there are some types that are more common than others, it is not possible to name all the kinds of oils and waxes that can be used. However, the two most used oils are obviously camellia oil and jojoba oil. These two types therefore allow an easy and durable treatment for your strings. They have little or no odor and generally do not cause skin irritation since they are compatible.

The most widely used wax is beeswax. It can be melted, then applied directly to the rope in small quantities to obtain resistance over time. Ideally, beeswax should be mixed with camellia oil for best results.

After a first application, it is always possible to repeat treatments afterwards. However, if you use the rope directly on human skin, you do not necessarily need to redo it. Although the effects of the oils or wax will gradually wear off, the rope will absorb the oil that is naturally produced by the skin. So, if you continue to use them, they preserve themselves.

To ensure the quality of your strings, it is recommended that you check them every year to ensure their condition and to determine whether it is necessary to re-treat or not.

Rope preparation

When you are new to rope, it is rare that you want to start by purchasing a roll of rope to prepare them yourself to your own specifications. You are more likely to buy some that are already ready to use. However, should you ever purchase some, there is an effective way to prepare your natural fiber ropes and allow you to build your own kit.

- We start by cutting the ropes to the lengths you want and making knots at the ends to prevent them from coming undone. The knot is as you wish, a simple knot is sufficient if it does not come off easily.

- Next, prepare a large pot of water and boil it. Once at the boil, we submerge the strings in it. This step brings out all the industrial oils that can be found on some strings on the market.

- To dry them, it is best to hang them out so that they are taut. Due to the water, they will tend to contract and lose length. When stretching them, make sure they are twisted enough, otherwise you will have to do this before stretching them.

- Once the strings are dry, use a low flame to quietly burn off any small fibers that may protrude from the string. It must be passed over the flame quickly enough that it cannot burn or even be damaged. You will probably need to iron two or three times for best results.

- Then, as was seen in the previous section, you will need to oil your strings to preserve them and that they can last you if possible. You can apply the oil to a cloth that you will slide over the ropes. If you do not put in enough, the protective effect will not be enough. If, on the other hand, you put too much of it, the rope will become oily and may stain fabrics that it may encounter.

Chapter 4

Why is there pleasure?

Shibari, and bondage more broadly, has become widely known through many references and different media. It has even become an important and widely recognized aspect of BDSM. What has caused this growth in popularity the most is the pleasure the restriction can bring. Both riggers and models can experience pleasure thanks to the Shibari. Usually, the reasons behind this pleasure are not the same for each of the two sides. So, if you are into Shibari or other forms of bondage in general, you will probably be motivated by the following points, but not necessarily. As much as this is a generalization that does not necessarily apply to everyone, there are certainly other grounds that concern you that will not be presented here. It should therefore be known that these are the most general and the most common which will be demonstrated.

So, while the reasons are different between riggers and models, there is a reason there will be a common source of fun. These are the physical contacts that will occur during the Shibari session. Oftentimes, this type of contact is done in a romantic relationship, but it is not always the case. Each situation is special and is different. It is therefore a way of exchanging contact with another person other than in a sexual way. Some cases also speak of an ability to communicate through the rope without having to speak openly. It is then possible to express oneself and share emotions and intentions through the rope.

There are undoubtedly similar points with both the tether and the tethered person, but as specified earlier, only the most common and frequently observed aspects will be discussed.

Model

There are several reasons why models get tied up repeatedly. Some of them have a particularly physical reason such as the sensations the rope provides when it encounters the body. Others involve a more psychological aspect such as an interest in the loss of freedom or in aesthetic pleasure.

The effect the strings have on the skin creates a sensation that influences the chemistry in the brain. When there is sudden pain, the brain releases adrenaline into the body that is meant to ease the pain and focus energy to prepare the body for a fight or flight. However, the constriction that is brought on by the cords is not sudden pain. Rather, it is a slower high that you can slowly get used to while still being bothersome and unusual for the body. The brain's response will then be to release other chemicals to soothe the pain but soothe and relax the body. In this way, the model can experience a generalized sense of well-being which may be like certain soft drugs. When a model is in an advanced state where the body has triggered great relaxation, the model may fall into a state often referred to as subspace. In this state, you must be more careful because the person is less conscious than usual.

In addition to losing mindfulness, there may also be a marked interest in the loss of freedom that comes from being attached. Since there is a strong restriction that limits some of the movements, actions, or gestures that one wants to make, one notices a strong decrease in freedom. It is not always a feeling that is appreciated, but with many models it is a goal to be achieved. As you lose your freedom, a feeling of being free outside your body sets in. This way the person can stop thinking about what is going on around them, what they can do or even forget about everything that is happening outside of the present moment. In this case, we focus on what is happening now. However, it is not a state that is necessarily easy to achieve. Getting there starts with not being in a stressful situation or with someone who makes us uncomfortable. If you can be relaxed from the start, you can more easily let go. You must therefore be in a state of confidence and have a certain inner calm to enjoy this experience that makes you want to start over.

A desire that can be sought from certain models is that of looking good, of beautifying themselves and of becoming the support of a work of art. Attractive designs give a sense of pride in being able to be highlighted by the rope while drawing the eye and attention to oneself. By having the ropes on you, you become the medium of art by becoming it yourself. Some riggers with a lot of experience even have a knack for being able to use the strings to highlight the physical advantages of the model while removing or hiding the flaws to make it a perfect piece.

It is up to you to ask yourself how it feels when you are attached and what your interests and intentions are. There are not necessarily wrong answers, the important thing is that you do it because you like it and it is not imposed or against your limits.

Rigger

The points that were put forward with the models do not apply directly to the riggers, but do indirectly, since they have the flip side. The sources of pleasure can therefore take its forms differently while resembling those of the models. The pursuit of giving pleasure to the partner, of having control over the other, or the pride of creating a piece of work using one person to create it are all popular and common points with riggers.

As you tie a person up, you can sometimes notice changes in facial expression. Whether it is grimaces from pain or a relaxation that appears in the face, it is quite a gratifying effect to know that one can be the cause and have control over the other. Some people have a natural urge to please others first and foremost, and that pleasure can be brought about by attaching someone. Thus, if the attached person will feel pleasure, the rigger will be able to feel just as much by the same fact.

By making such a large restriction, the model may no longer be able to move. With the rigger, this translates into a higher sense of power since he has direct control over the person. By being in control of the session, the burden of responsibility becomes more important, since you must be responsible for yourself, but also for another person and the rope to know what to do with them. This overload of responsibility can bring about a state of confidence and satisfaction that makes us feel more powerful than usual. This state is commonly called domspace. This is often the reverse state to subspace that is often experienced by riggers. When a person offers us his confidence so that we can make his body an artistic creation to attach it as we want, the feeling of power becomes even more important.

Much like an artist proud of his work, the rigger can enjoy creating a work from the rope on someone's body. In this way, it can be exhibited, whether through photography, video or even in public performance. Even if it is not shown publicly, since the subject can sometimes be taboo, there will always be pride in knowing what we create and what we are capable of. This feeling is reinforced when one goes beyond one's own limits by succeeding in creating increasingly complex and aesthetically improving patterns.

Again, your main sources of pleasure may not be among these points. These are the most common reasons, but there can be an infinite number of them. The important thing is to do it for the right reasons without trying to hurt or go against anyone's limits.

Chapter 5

Safety issues

It is obvious that many accidents have happened due to bad practices or mistakes that have been made. A simple search on the Internet can see how common they can be. The goal here is not to scare and discourage doing it, but rather to force a little awareness of the risks to prevent them and to know how to act to prevent them from occurring.

Selection of the body parts to tie

Not all parts of the body can be attached. Some areas are more sensitive than others and can cause short- or long-term damage. Generally, one wants to avoid any areas that could cut off the flow of blood or crush a nerve. Other parts may be discouraged just to avoid discomfort.

The areas to avoid are:

- The neck

Obviously, many nerves, arteries and veins pass through the neck. You should therefore avoid the entire neck region as much as possible. Even if the cords do not pass near the nerves and arteries, there is also the risk of suffocation.

- The brachial plexus

There is a nerve in the armpits that can cause discomfort as well as compression. You must therefore avoid tying a knot or putting too much tension.

- The radial nerve

It is located slightly hidden between the triceps and the deltoid. The exact point to avoid varies from person to person. To find it, just feel the area, asking your partner to mention when there is any discomfort. A lot of times when starting out you never put ropes in this area as it is one of the most common causes of accidents.

- Inside the elbow

If you put too much tension on the inside of the elbow, you cross the ulnar nerve, which can also be compressed.

- The wrists

The median nerve passes through the wrists. When attaching at this level, you should never over-tighten.

- groin

Between the pubis and the upper inner thigh is the obturator nerve which is tender and where no knots should be placed.

- Knees

Near the knees, the saphenous and peroneal nerves prevent significant tension. In addition, when the leg is extended, the kneecap can move more freely requiring more care.

- Ankles

The peroneal nerve ends at the level of the foot passing through the ankle. The same precautions as for the wrists apply.

How to avoid injuries

All kinds of injuries can occur, and it is as much the responsibility of the rigger as the model to ensure safety during the session. The rigger must make sure that everything goes smoothly. The human also has its limits. He also cannot know the exact state of mind of the model. For this reason, the model must take charge of its own safety by being attentive to what is going on. It should not be taken for granted that the rigger is aware of every discomfort and it should be mentioned.

The best way to communicate the state of a situation is through a color code commonly called safe words. Yellow is to indicate discomfort, a situation to be corrected or to ask for a little time to adjust to a new position. Red indicates the intention to stop the session for any reason. Once spoken, the rigger is obligated to start detaching the model to put it in a stable situation to help it feel better.

- The falls

One of the most common, but most often underestimated, causes of accidents is a fall. Whether caused by a lack of balance with the model's hands tied behind her back or a rope breaking during a suspension, impact on the ground is never pleasant. It sounds mundane, but it happens frequently enough that it is a concern to pay attention to.

The easiest way to prevent this type of accident is to provide a soft surface for practicing. Whether it is a foam mat, blankets, or a mattress, falling on it will be much more pleasant than falling to the ground directly.

In the event of a suspension, it is essential to check your equipment to make sure there is no possible damage. A slightly cracked carabiner or a rope starting to unravel are signs of impending danger.

- Nerve compressions

Injuries from nerve compressions are not to be taken lightly. As was mentioned earlier, there are several tender points on the body that one should be extra careful with. Signs of nerve compression will usually be felt in the extremities, such as the fingers or toes.

Feelings can vary from person to person when this happens. There may be tingling, numbness, feeling hot or cold, etc. When it is not usual, it is not a good sign and the situation needs to be restored quickly.

This is a risk that can happen very quickly. From the first moments, after-effects can begin to appear. One of the first symptoms that can happen is loss of sensitivity in your fingertips. If nerve compression is neglected, this loss can be felt days or even weeks after the session. In more extreme cases, it might never come back.

There are several ways that the rigger can check the state of model members. For the fingers, for example, it is possible to grab the hand and ask the model to shake the hand of the rigger. By judging by the grip strength, one can assess the risk. If both hands are busy, the rigger can ask to make shapes with the hands that require all the muscles to contract. A deformed or weak-looking face is a risk that needs to be addressed.

The model, also responsible for her own safety, can use her thumb to touch the tips of all other fingers at a frequency of every 2 to 5 minutes to check for any numbness.

If you are in the presence of nerve compression, several solutions exist. As the case is advanced, the best solution is to stop the session and first detach the ropes that compress the numb areas. Extreme cases involve cutting the rope with a scissors or other tool specially designed for this use. Otherwise, if the situation allows, it is sufficient to move the ropes slightly to a less risky area or to loosen so that there is less pressure on the nerves.

- Blood circulation

When a limb is strongly compressed to the point that the skin begins to change color, there is a lack of blood circulation. Aside from the color, we can also witness it by noting a decrease in temperature. In this kind of situation, it is not necessarily catastrophic, especially when the limbs are quite massive like the thighs. The veins that pass through them are large enough to support the flow of blood when the cords are detached. The main risk that can be hidden, especially in the forearms or calves, is nerve compression that occurs at the same time.

- Rope burns

By pulling on a rope, friction can occur in contact with the skin. When pulled quickly, the friction can cause a burn which can be particularly painful. Unless you are a masochist and have been negotiated in advance, this is not a very pleasant experience to have. Plastic fiber ropes more easily cause these burns.

The easiest way is to handle the rope calmly and to avoid large sudden movements by pulling the rope. Extra care should be taken when the rope enters between two limbs which are close together and which exerts pressure on the rope.

- Nausea, fainting

If the model does not feel well or has symptoms of unconsciousness or nausea, your best bet from this point on is to start detaching it and putting it in a stable situation. Being restricted can be a taxing experience on the body, and sometimes it does not take much to make you feel unwell.

Knowing the cause of this condition is the best way to bring a situation back to normal. It could be dehydration, too much heat, or a drop in pressure. This is usually the rarest case of risk, but one that should not be overlooked and always be aware that it can happen at one time or another.

Instruction for rope play

As a rigger or a model, there are many things you need to keep in mind to have a fun and safe session for everyone. Some are more rigger oriented while others are more model oriented. Regardless of which side you consider yourself to be on, it is relevant to know both sides of the coin. This will then let you know what aspects the other is focusing on and putting importance on.

For both

A first aspect to consider and which forms the basis of all interactions, in the world of bondage or not, is communication. The point is not to give advice on how to improve your interactions in this part, but to bring up points that bother you or interest you with your partner. It takes place before, during and after the session.

Before you start to tie up, and especially if this is your first meeting with this person, you need to negotiate. The negotiation is about finding common ground mainly on what you want to do during the said session, if there are any physical restrictions or health problems and the limits not to cross. Safe words can also be set up there for security. By establishing these few rules, it helps to avoid situations that could make us uncomfortable or hurt us. It is essential that each partner is aware of the dangers that there may be and how to overcome them. It depends on the experience of each and the equipment available to be ready for anything.

During the session, do not hesitate to share our concerns or discomfort. It is not a failure if our partner pronounces the safe word. You are not a bad role model if you use it. It allows you to see a possible mistake or avoid a situation that could get worse.

In the end, a retrospection helps to highlight what went well and what can be improved for next time. Comments should not always be taken personally. Especially in the beginnings you will have a lot to learn and practice. Sometimes you must know how to silence your ego and consider the constructive comments that will allow you to become a better rigger.

You are both responsible for the security of the session. You should never assume that the other is taking care of everything. If you are not feeling well, would like to change something that was not planned, or wish to quit, it is your responsibility to say so, the other cannot guess.

Make sure you are in a state that allows you to be alert and ready to respond. Therefore, avoid playing when you are tired, sick, or under the influence of drugs or medication. Alcohol can help you relax and feel comfortable, but it also reduces judgment and alters perceptions. While it is not recommended to take it during a session, you should rely on your own judgment to know what is right and wrong to do.

Rigger

You will oversee the session that will take place. Prepare accordingly by having everything you need to avoid unnecessary risks. Always remember to have a sharp object to cut the strings if necessary. For sessions including sensualism, sensory deprivation or psychological games, provide a blindfold to hide the eyes. Make sure you have the necessary number of cords of the correct length, width, and type of fibers that you need.

More extreme games including fire, candles, blades or whatever else you can imagine requires additional needs and materials. You will therefore need a fire extinguisher, a first aid kit, etc. Always be prepared for whatever you plan to do.

If you do not have a clear idea of what to do and how to go about it, it is always better to plan more than not enough. The session can be improvised, not the preparation. You just need to have a bag on hand with all the equipment ready to use to be ready for a session at any time.

Be ready to intervene and know what to do for the riskiest scenarios such as a power failure, an emergency evacuation, a health problem, etc.

You should never exceed your capabilities too much. Obviously, we must try to surpass ourselves by trying new things that are more and more advanced, but that should not be beyond what is possible for us. There is a big difference between what you want to do and what you can do.

If you are in any doubt whether you can do something that is potentially dangerous, it is best to have someone nearby with more experience to guide you and intervene if necessary.

When working with someone you have never played before, it is also best to take it slow at the start, so you get to know the model's body better, their reactions, their abilities, etc.

Like your own abilities, you should not exceed the capabilities of the model either. For a pleasant session, never put your model in danger or in a situation that could put them outside their comfort zone, both physically and mentally. No matter how much you want to try something, if your model does not, there is no way it will happen.

A mistake you should never make is to leave a model unsupervised. Many accidents have happened this way and could have been avoided. To give the impression of being left alone without being, you can get a monitor to watch babies while they sleep. This way you can leave the room while keeping an eye on the attached person.

ModelsWhen starting out as a model, it can be difficult to know if a rigger is experienced or not. You must be on your guard when it comes to whether you can be trusted. Ideally, the first few times should be in a dungeon or Shibari dojo to have an audience around to make sure everything runs smoothly. In a more private setting, it may be enough to ask a friend to monitor remotely or to exchange text messages with to make sure everything is fine.

Just because someone seems to know the subject, has a lot of equipment, or claims to have taken courses (online or in real life) does not mean that they know what they are doing. It is always best to rely on references that can be provided to validate that the person is acting in a safe manner.

Make sure you state your intentions and expectations to the rigger and that there are no misunderstandings. Many problematic situations can be avoided by following this one tip. The same goes for any medical condition that requires special attention.

Above all, do not assume that the rigger oversees everything. It is a lot to deal with as a situation and even the slightest hint about your safety or comfort is a big help that may just make the experience better.

Aftercare

A workout can sometimes be a strain on the body in terms of exertion. Especially for the model who sometimes must undergo unusual tensions and restrictions that can overwhelm the muscles and even impose awkward positions. As the body quickly depletes its resources, like a sporting effort, in energy and water, it is sometimes necessary to refuel after a session.

Aftercare is a term that comes from BDSM meaning to get back to normal. It is therefore, as much for the rigger as the model of a moment to come back down to earth after a session. It is even more important when one or both partners have reached domspace or subspace. The euphoria of the moment is far from reality and you need to allow yourself some time for the effect to wear off and sometimes just work normally.

Getting back to normal is all about knowing what you need to make yourself feel good and what you need. It might as well be a little rest, comfort, or sticking with someone. If there has been sweating or rather intense physical exertion, intake of sugars or water may be necessary. It is up to you to tell your partner what you need.

Aftercare and the benefits it can bring should not be taken too lightly. This is an essential step for the smooth running of a session. Thus, psychologically, the person can feel more secure and in a more receptive state. Trust is established more easily, and it helps to strengthen bonds. It therefore also makes it possible to give a positive experience while making it possible to encourage a next session later.

CHAPTER 6

Basic Ties

Single column tie

The simple column tie is especially useful for creating a first anchor point which will then be used to do whatever you want. We can then start on anything that acts as a single column, such as a wrist, an ankle, or a chair leg. There are a multitude of ways to make one. Here is an example of making it quick and easy to run.

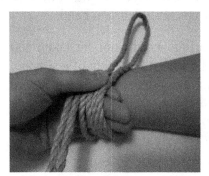

1. To start tying a simple column knot, you must first start with the bight. We will first start by making two full turns of the column without crossing the ropes. As explained previously, there are certain sensitive areas where nerves can pass. For this reason, we do not want the knot to be too tight.

To leave a secure lousse, you should leave your fingers between the rope and the spine to keep space.

2. Ideally, we will try to have a remaining bight of about 4 to 5 inches. If it is shorter, it can be difficult to complete the knot and lose resistance. If it is longer it can be more difficult to work with and

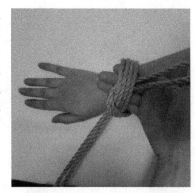

becomes a waste of rope. We then pass the bight over the two turns we made, then below.

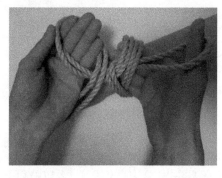

3.   On the longer side of the rope, we will create a loop whose tail will be blocked on both sides by the rope. Otherwise, if it has a free side, the knot will not hold. The easiest way to do this is to twist your wrist a bit as shown in the photo to grab the rope before returning your hand to its original position.

4.   The bight will then have to pass through the loop that we have just created. Keep the tension in the bight while pulling on the string to reduce the size of the loop. This tension breaks the noose that is the loop. Without it, the rope would start to tighten the spine which can cause pain.

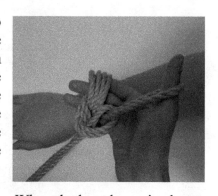

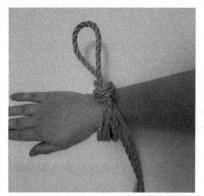

5.   When the knot has seized, you can remove your fingers and hold the bight with one hand and the rest of the rope with the other and exert force in opposite directions. It may be necessary to pull harder on one side and then the other alternately to achieve some stability.

This is an extremely popular and one of the most used basic ties, especially when starting out. We should not hesitate to practice repeatedly to obtain muscle memory that allows us to be able to do it without even having to think about it.

When you feel comfortable, you can afford to do it all with one hand (no matter which side) or even with your eyes closed.

Double column tie

The double column knot is quite common and very frequently used. Indeed, it can be used as handcuffs, to restrict or for a possible complete immobilization.

The advantage of this knot is that it allows to tie two parts together. It can then be used to handcuff someone in the case of two wrists but can also be used to attach a wrist to a fixed bar to prevent movement.

Much like the simple column tie, there is a wide variety and techniques to achieve this restriction. Ideally, you would find a way unique to yourself that best represents your style, but here is an example to build a basis.

It is better to have the two parts closer together than in the following example so that the wrists cannot come out of the loops. The photos simply make it easier to visualize the instructions. You can also space it out on your first few times to practice and feel comfortable.

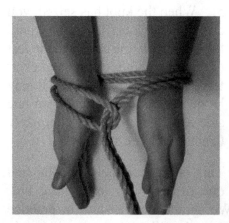

1.   We start by circling the two columns using a rope and passing the rope flow through the bight to form a loop. Preferably, the bight and the rope flow are side by side which makes it possible to be equal between the two strands. This small turn allows for easy gliding if turning one way but locks out completely if turning the other way. You can try it for yourself to better understand the benefits this little tour can bring you.

2. By folding the rope in the other direction, thus blocking the rope, we will form another full turn around the two columns to pass again through the ropes to form a new loop. This time around, we do not want to put it through the bight like the first, but through the fold that we formed in the previous step.

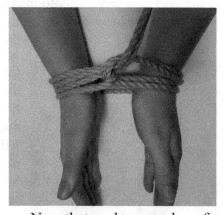

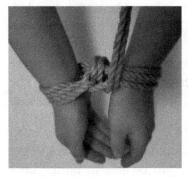

3. Now that we have our base for the knot, we will isolate the two columns from each other which will prevent slipping out of the links. To do this, we will simply start by taking the rope flow that we have and pass it directly between the two columns, making a full turn of all the ropes that we have already placed so far. The rope flow must end at the starting point of this loop. By putting tension on this loop, we can see that the large loop encircling the columns narrows in its center. It is thanks to this trick that the wrists or ankles cannot come out after the knot is finished.

4. This step is like the previous one, but in a smaller version. With the rope flow we have left, we will pass it between the ropes of the front stage loop and the side of the first column. We will therefore try to walk along this column over its entire length, then come back in the same way in the opposite direction to the side of the second column. We have now come to circle the loop that had just been made

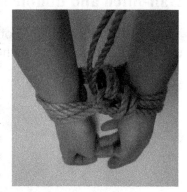

27

in the previous step. This loop will reinforce the middle loop and allow the outer loop to be better maintained.

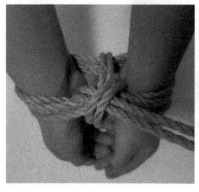

5.   The knot is complete and holds the two columns together but leaving a space. This knot should be finished by fixing it so that it does not come off. To get there, we will slowly loosen the last loop we made. We will pass the rope flow between the middle loop and the origin of the previous loop. About the same place where step 3 ended. Once the rope has passed through space, you can apply tension to tighten the loop. Here it is a case of a tension knot. The greater the tension on the rope flow, the more the loop will tighten, putting more pressure on the rope flow. The tension exerted allows the knot to hold. When you take that tension away, it easily loosens.

It may seem complex at first glance and may take a few tries to get there. This is a matter of practice. You will be able to tie the knot closer and closer with each attempt to create a handcuff that is not easily released. Be careful not to make it too tight, especially at the wrists and ankles where there may be compression.

Half-hitch and double half hitch

The half-hitch is a small knot of friction that can come undone very easily, but which holds if there is tension in the rope flow. It can

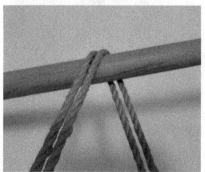

then be used to quickly create a blockage so that one rope does not slip unintentionally over another. Its implementation is fast and quite efficient.

1. When a rope line is already established, it may be thinkable to just want to place the rope over it so that you have a fulcrum as shown in the photo. If you do it on your own, you will notice that the point of intersection between the two strings can easily slide over each other. Which is not what we are looking to do here.

2. To put it in place, we will first want to put a small twist on it which will ensure greater friction. To do this, when the rope has passed over the rope line already in place, we will bring the rope back in the direction of its point of origin.

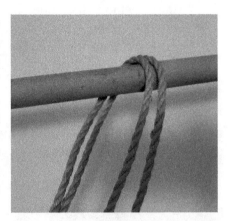

3. Before returning to the direction you want to go, you will pass the rope so that it is blocked by the one you just placed in the previous step. You can then experience for yourself that when trying to change the intersection of places, it is much more difficult when tension is exerted in the rope flow.

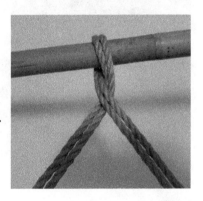

The double half hitch uses the same principle but makes sure that it is more stable and that it does not come undone on its own when there is no tension. This knot is most often used in a hanging context where you do not want the knot that holds the hanging line to come off, which could result in a fall.

1. To do this, we will start with the half hitch that we did previously, which we will repeat the step, but in reverse. This means that if the rope goes first in front, then behind the line in place, then the second will go back, then forward. By alternating the direction of

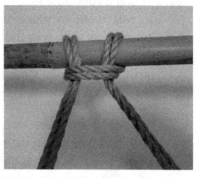

the knot, effective blocking is ensured in both directions.

If you use a plastic fiber rope, the friction will be less effective, so more will probably have to be done to get a tie that will not come off.

Various Styles of friction

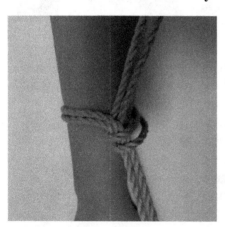

There are several ways to set up a friction knot that is intended to hold the strings together. Traditionally, conventional knots are not tolerated, which is why friction knots are of particular importance. It is not just any knot that is suitable for every situation. It also depends on your personal style and the aesthetic you want to give it.

There are a multitude of friction knots and each has variations to create a wide range that can enrich your creations. It is therefore obvious that it will not be possible to cover them all in this short guide, but three will be presented that can serve as a basis for your beginnings.

Figure 8 friction

1. To put this friction knot in place, we start making a loop around a limb around which we want to create an attachment point. At the point where the two parts of the rope meet, we will make them cross by aligning them each in an opposite direction.

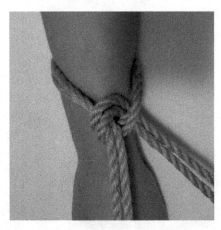

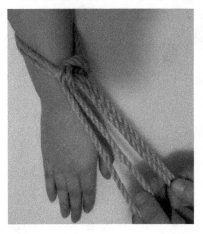

2. The part of the rope that includes the bight will go over the rope surrounding the limb returning to its original direction. At this point, the bight and the rope flow are parallel to each other.

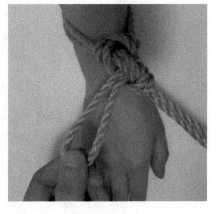

3. Bring the bight back over the knot we have already mounted so far and then pass it through behind the limb loop to direct the bight down, again, parallel to the rope flow.

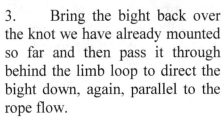

4. We will finally set up a half hitch with the rope flow to keep the bight in place. We will then make the loop around the rope flow and pass the bight again through the formed space. We will then be able to tighten the knot so that it stays in place. It is important to make sure the friction knot is tight. The rope flow and loop are

linked and can quickly become a noose if the knot is not secured and prevents it from slipping.

Cross friction

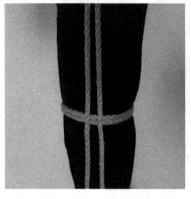

1. To be able to use the cross-friction knot, we must obviously have strings that form an " X " and where the friction will be placed at the intersection so that there is no friction. against each other. While a first rope is already in place, the knot is built by installing the rope perpendicular. It must therefore pass over or under the one already present. In this example, it will be on top.

2. We then take the rope flow to make a U-turn which will pass below the line in place to return to the original direction.

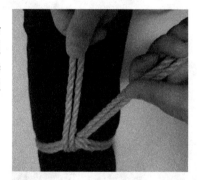

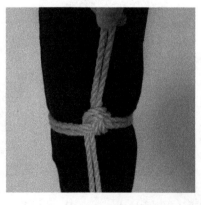

3. Finally, the rope flow will pass over the part just placed, then under the perpendicular rope. By putting tension on the rope flow, the knot is held in place and stabilized. You can then continue to use the rope without worrying about unwanted movement.

Obviously, from an aesthetic point of view, it is possible to adapt it as much as desired by alternating only the directions if the basic structure of the knot is respected.

Twisted cross friction

This friction knot is like the previous one. The only difference is to give an overview that it was placed starting from the other direction.

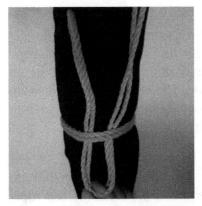

1. We start again with two parallel lines of strings. The difference with the previous knot begins by not passing the rope flow directly below, but only a part that will form a loop below the line already in place.

2. The rope flow will then pass through this loop, passing over the perpendicular rope to surround it. By applying tension, we find ourselves in the same situation as the previous knot except that it is in the opposite direction. Once again, continuous voltage must be applied to keep it in place.

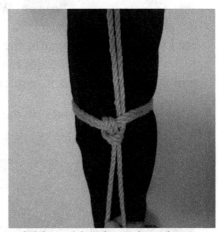

Connecting ropes

As it was mentioned at the beginning of this guide, the strings have different lengths, and it is necessary to make connections between each string to continue to make a more complex assembly than using a single string. As you can imagine, there are again several ways to connect your strings together. Only three examples will be presented that are the most frequently mentioned, but nothing prevents you from discovering more on your own or from other sources.

Lark's head

This technique is the simplest of all. It is fast and most often it is tailored to what you want to do. To be able to use it, however, you must have a knot at the ends of your ropes. If your ends are smooth and only held by a string to prevent them from fraying, you will not be able to use this technique.

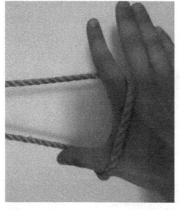

1.   We start by making a double loop with the bight of the new rope that we want to take to serve as an extension. The best way to do this is to slide your thumb and forefinger into the bight.

2.   Then stick the ends of the thumb and forefinger together to encircle the two strands of the rope. We lowered the bight which rested on the back of the hand towards the rope flow. We then obtain a double loop which has the bight as its center.

3.   Collect the ends of the rope

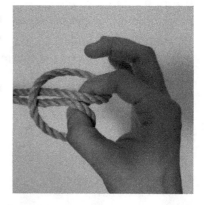

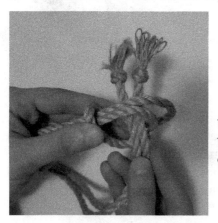

that you want to extend and slip them into the double loop obtained in the previous step.

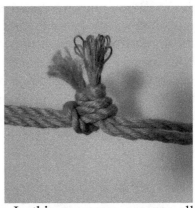

4. The double loop is tightened around the ends. You can then use the end knots to act as a stopper so that the new rope does not slip and come loose.

Square knot

This knot is much the same as the previous one, but there are a few more steps to provide more benefits. In this case, you can use all kinds of ropes, with or without knots at the ends. It can also be used at any length and not just at the ends of the rope which makes it a strategic extension.

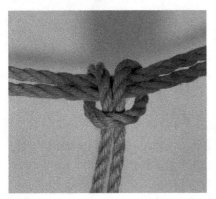

1. Starting with the previous knot, in this case we can afford to start somewhere other than the ends.

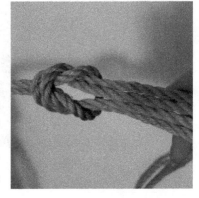

2. On one side of the knot, there is a space between the two ropes, the opposite of where the rope flow is. By spacing the two loops apart, they can be made to slide along the rope which must be extended. It will therefore be folded in half, folded back on itself.

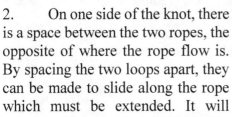

3.   By pulling on both sides, on one side, the four strands of the folded rope and on the other, both new ropes, we exert a tension that will allow the knot to be fixed. We can then continue to tie from this new rope while maintaining tension with it.

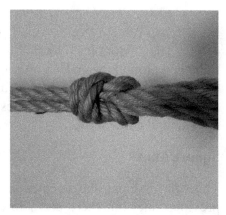

Sheet bend

This technique is used less regularly but can be useful when you have a rope with low friction. It is a simple knot around the bight to secure it and keep it in place.

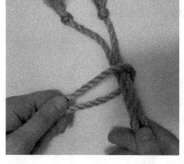

1. Pass the ends of the extended string inside the bight.

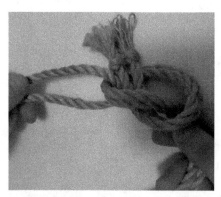

2.We use the ends to then circle the rope flow of the new rope and pass it through the loop we just created.

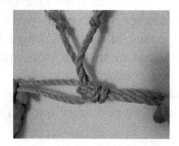

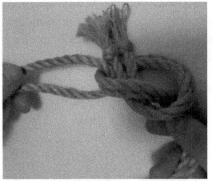

3.   You can finish by applying tension to complete the knot by pulling the rope flow of the new rope and the old rope while making sure that the ends stay in place.

Cat's pawn

This technique is not really a knot but can be very quick and easy to do in an erotic setting where you need to hang on when the hands are tied.

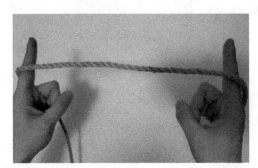

1. Take a section of a strand of rope using both index fingers where the rope is simply resting on them.

2.   We begin to make a loop on each side with each index. With the string in front of you, the left hand moves counterclockwise, while the right hand goes clockwise.

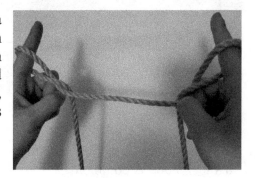

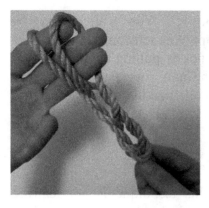

3.   Repeat the previous step two to three more times to accumulate the curls. The two sides are then folded over one another.

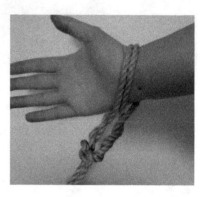

4.   We are going to widen the loops in which the index fingers were wide enough to fit a hand.

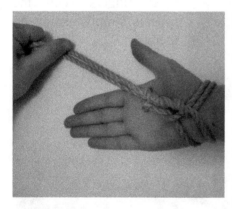

5.   We will direct the twisted rope towards the side of the palm where we can slide the rope from the outside to the inside of the palm to tighten the rope around the wrist thus preventing the hand from being able to come out.

By holding the hand in this way, the restriction is present, but it is important that the person hold the rope in their hand to avoid causing nerve compression in the wrist.

Chain braiding

This technique is commonly referred to as "Daisy Chain" and is a kind of leash that allows a large amount of rope to be stored in a smaller space easily. Its main advantage is being able to undo almost instantly and without difficulty. It is therefore particularly useful for storing rope in an aesthetic way, but also for making a leash with someone, since it does not come undone until it is unlocked.

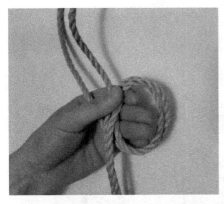

1. Starting with the bight, keep a small distance that will not be used. In some cases, this short distance can be for tethered and have an anchor point. We then form a small loop.

2. Half pass the rope flow through the loop so that only part of the rope passes through. Then pull both the one-way bight and the rope flow through the loop to reduce the size of the loop. For best results, do not pull until the knot is completely restricted. It is better if it is a little relaxed.

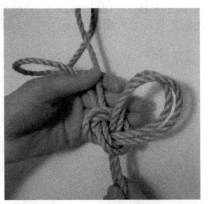

3. A new loop has formed, and we pass part of the rope flow through it again, then pull on both ends to form a second link in the chain.

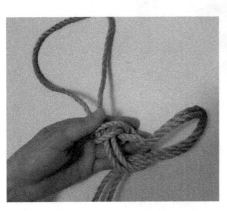

4. Continue to follow these steps until the rope is completely used or until the desired length is reached.

5. Finally, we want to block the chain to prevent it from completely undoing itself. To do this, we

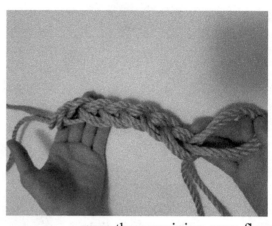

pass the remaining rope flow through the last loop completely created. The ends of the rope are then pulled, and the chain formed so far. This last link will block the rope. To undo it, all you must do is remove this part of the rope and pull on it.

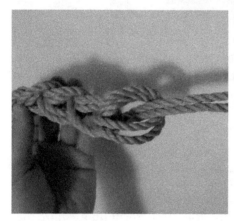

Chapter 7

Chest harness

There are several types of harnesses. Some have a practical function that allows them to be strong and not hurt during a suspension for example, others are very much focused on aesthetics. There are also some that have for primary purpose to live a sensual experience and awaken the senses of the model. Obviously, it is quite possible to combine several of its characteristics at the same time. Simply, when you start out, you better have an idea of what you are trying to achieve as a result to have a plan of action established.

Pentagram

This harness, basically, is not made for suspension unless you upgrade it to be. It clearly has an aesthetic purpose and by modifying it, we can offer it several different styles.

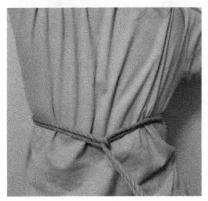

1. We start by making a first waist measurement from the back where the rope flow will pass inside the bight, then move in the opposite direction like the first steps of the double column tie. Going through the front of the body, the rope is placed directly under the chest.

2. By forming the second turn, this time, the rope passes over the chest, then the rope flow will pass through the previous fold formed by the bight. We will then direct the rope flow towards the shoulder, making almost a U-turn.

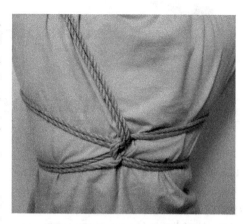

3. The rope will slide along the shoulder to between the

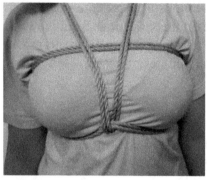

breasts, passing through the collarbone where we will form a "V" with the lower rope line, then do the opposite way going towards the second shoulder.

4. Back in the back, we will pass the rope flow through one of the folds of the central node to move towards a flank by performing a

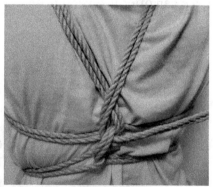

U-turn as much as possible. There are always two options when orienting the rope flow, either to the left or to the right. To ensure better hold, the fold should be as pronounced as possible to obtain greater friction between the strings.

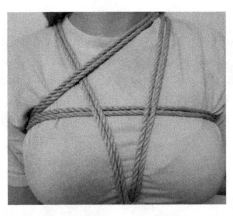

5. The rope flow should go to the shoulder furthest from the coming flank without putting too much tension as we pass near the neck and arteries.

6. Repeat the same operation as in the previous two steps to reproduce the same pattern symmetrically from side to side.

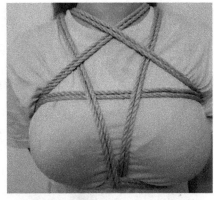

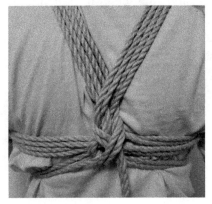

7. The remaining rope flow can finally be used to lock at the center knot using a friction knot to hold everything in place.

Variation:

Although in this case the changes can be rather subtle, they can still reflect your own style. Every detail can be important. For a more classic finish, we can alternate the rope that we pass forming the pentagram once above, then below the others creating a more symmetrical overview in general.

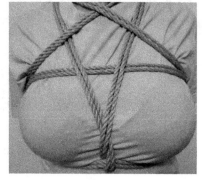

You can also replace the "V" in step 3 with a half hitch to better hold the shape in place and prevent slipping.

Shinju

While not as extravagant as the pentagram, this harness offers better stability and strength that may allow it to better set up other patterns later. This is a standard and commonly used harness that will come in handy on many occasions.

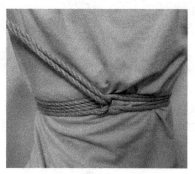

1. The harness begins by making two turns around the torso, the ropes of which pass directly under the chest and the central attachment point in the middle of the back, following the same method as the first two steps of the double column tie.

2. Still following the same principle as before, we go around the torso twice again, but this time the strings will be located directly above the chest, parallel to that placed in step 1. The rope flow can then be oriented towards one of the two shoulders.

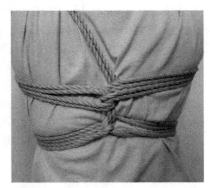

3. The rope flow will descend

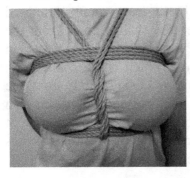

between the breasts to make a half hitch, then make a full turn around the rope just turned around before returning to the opposite shoulder.

4. Towards the central knot, a friction knot can be made to keep the harness stable without it being able

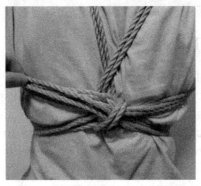

to come undone.

Variations:

The possibilities for variations are more varied for the Shinju harness and adapt better depending on the situation and what you want to do.

A first option consists in not

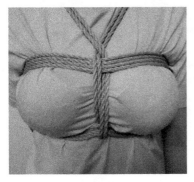

making the half hitch at the height of the lower line, but rather at that of the upper line, thus creating two lines parallel to the vertical. This case also changes its name and is better known under the term of "bikini harness".

Another option is to alternate the upper and lower breast lines to cross between the breasts. The result is a harness with a more refined look, but a little less resistant and comfortable. There is then no possibility of putting the V connecting towards the shoulders.

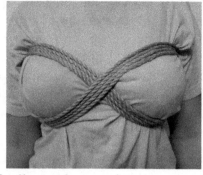

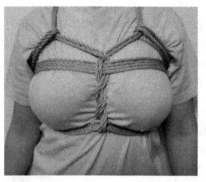

Finally, a last variant proposed moves the strings away from the neck forming the "V" to prevent slipping which could cause pain. By simply using hitch from the rear and pulling the strings in question towards the flanks, it widens and increases its stability as the tension increases.

Takate Kote

This harness is one of the most popular and can be found in many contexts, especially when suspended thanks to its very stable structure. It also helps to keep the arms fixed and provide greater control. Since it is necessary to tie up near certain areas at risk of nerve compression, it is best to have already practiced other harnesses before starting this one. It is also called a "box tie" because of the box shape formed by the arms.

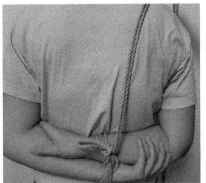

1. The harness begins by holding the hands together behind the back. Ideally, the two forearms meet so that the hands touch the elbows. If your model is not flexible enough to be able to do this, at least both wrists should be able to be aligned. Both wrists should face each other and not expose the inside of a wrist. This then avoids a possible nerve compression. Around the wrists or forearms, you must make a single column tie with the rope flow oriented towards the upper body.

2. Next, complete two full turns of the torso, including the arms. In the torso, this first line is located just above the chest, while in the arms, it is just above the sensitive area of the radial nerve. In general, the rope should cover half the fold of the armpit. After the second round, we will make a

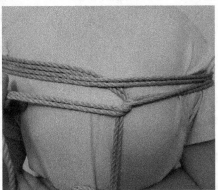

fold with the rope connecting with the wrists. Obviously, we make sure to center this fold towards the spine.

3. At this point, the ropes can be adjusted to distribute the tension so that it is even on each side of the arms and between the two ropes. The best way to do this is to slip a finger between the arm and the string and slide it across the surface. If the finger slips too easily, the string is not tight enough. If, on the contrary, the finger passes with difficulty or can hurt your model, the string is too tight. In both cases, the tension will have to be adjusted.

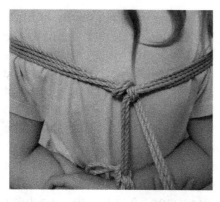

4. When the tension in the rope is adequate, we must block this first step of the TK. To achieve this, we pass the rope flow which has folded over the line already in place to pass it behind it to encircle all the ropes. This then allows all of them to be blocked and not just a few.

5. To complete this friction knot, repeat the same step as the previous one, but on the other side. So, we send the rope opposite the knot in front and up, then pass it behind all the ropes again.

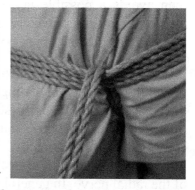

6. The rope flow will then slide between the arm and the torso to encircle the line of rope at the front of the body. This should go from top to bottom and not the other way around when it encircles this line. You should not put too much tension on it either, but enough to keep it going.

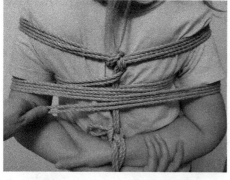

7. Going back to the back of the body, we move towards the other arm where we will repeat the same step.

8. We then perform for the second time, two turns of the torso including the arms. This time the ropes will be below the chest and pass between the radial nerve area and the elbow at the arm. We therefore repeat step 2 at a different height.

9. We will check the tension again by running a finger between the strings and the arm, making sure that it is neither too tight nor not enough. We can then adjust the tension before blocking them.

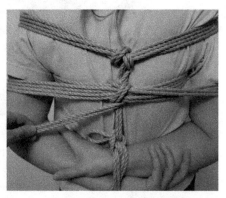

10. Once the two turns are done, we can again tie a friction knot as in step 4 and 5 to lock the rope turns as well as the ropes that we placed in steps 6 and 5. 7. This time, by blocking them, we will then take all the strings that are free and not framed.

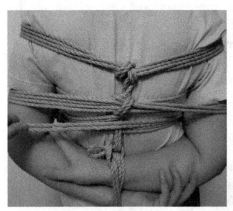

11. Once this friction knot is established, we can then use the rope flow to repeat steps 6 and 7 to block the second row of ropes that have been put on. Always passing between the arm and the torso and circling it from top to bottom. We can go to the other side to do the same on the other arm.

12. Finally, with what is left of the rope flow, it can be used to block near the center knot with a friction knot to hold everything together one last time.

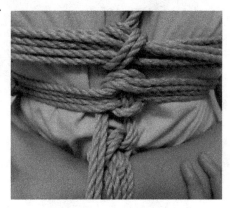

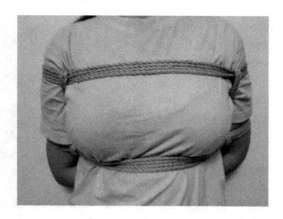

Variations:

We can add the option of putting the same "V" as we find in the examples of Shinju to obtain more support, especially at the shoulders. So, you can put a V like the one made at the beginning of the pentagram, a crossed V, a twisted V, a combination of these, or other alternatives you can imagine. This type of variant will make it possible to offer greater support and distribute part of the load on the shoulders, as in the case of a suspension, for example. You must be careful, however, because variants including a V can bring strings tight near the neck and where more attention should be paid.

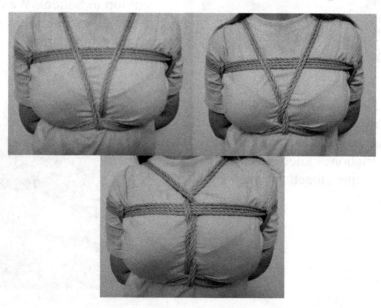

Another common variation is to run ropes running from the sides to the shoulders that are on the same side and repeat this step on each side. To prevent them from slipping out, we add a last string from side to side, encircling the two ropes just added to keep them

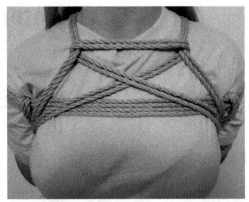

close together. Thanks to this technique, we continue to keep the stability that we find with the V-variants. As the natural state of this arrangement is to slide outwards, the risks of the strings coming closer to the neck are lower. However, you must be careful because the risk is still present.

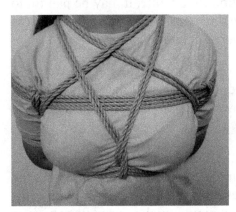

Finally, by remaining creative, we can even form a kind of pentagram to add the aesthetic aspect. The central V acts in the same way as the variant seen previously. The two extra strings do not add anything special that could be technically useful. If you like the pentagram style, you will surely want to include it.

Chapter 8

Others

Futomomo

Futomomo is a restriction technique that is done in the legs. It therefore allows a blocking folding the leg on itself preventing it from unfolding. Since this is a large member, you can afford to exert a great deal of tension on the ropes, but that is no reason to diminish alertness. However, it is not recommended to leave one leg with a Futomomo for a long period of time, which could cause numbness. When the leg is left in this position for a while, it may be painful to straighten the leg after loosening the ropes. So be sure to take it slow to get the leg used to returning to its natural position.

There are many ways to make one, from the simplest to the most complex and extravagant. The one that will be shown is not necessarily the simplest but allows the leg to be firmly held in place and by exerting great tension in it.

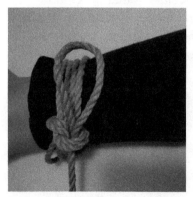

1. A Futomomo begins by making a single column tie at the ankle. As the tension will be high with this technique, make sure you have a comfortable space between the buckle and the ankle to avoid nerve compression.

2. Keeping the same height as the single column tie, make two full turns of the leg folded over on itself. To avoid a point of compression, we arrange for all the strings to be parallel and stick to each other. If one rope were passed over another, pain could be caused as the tension increases.

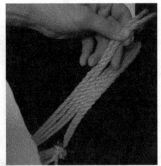

3. When the two turns are done and the rope flow is side by side with the starting loop, a second double turn is formed by bringing

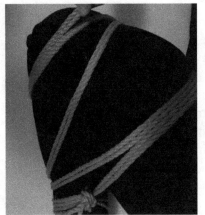

the rope closer to the knee. At the crease at the back of the knee, we visualize an imaginary line going from the front of the leg to the thigh. The rope flow that we are going to place will have to lie on this imaginary line. You can then do the two full laps there in the same way as in the previous step. In doing these, you must be more careful and go more delicately. As you move closer to the knee, the strings will tend to want to slide toward the knee when tension is applied.

4. After both turns are done, we run our finger between the leg and the strings, going from top to bottom. We pass the rope flow between the leg and the finger, then we pass it over the line of rope freshly put in place. We then use our fingers to grab the rope flow.

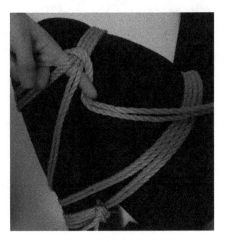

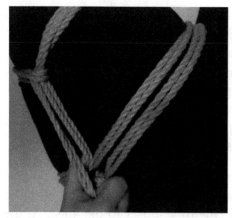

5. By pulling out the rope flow with our finger, we will bring it as close as possible to the center, towards the fold between the thigh and the calf. We will then block this point with the rope flow by exerting a downward tension perpendicular to the two lines of ropes.

6. We will replace the rope that already united the two lines of ropes so that it is also perpendicular. It may be too tense to be able to move it. To do so, we will then add tension on the second turn of the second step to have enough play to bring the rope in question where we want to put it, parallel to the one coming from the top.

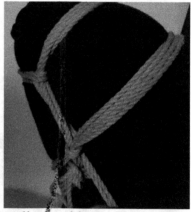

7. The rope flow will circle the bottom line making a U-turn. To block the other rope, we will pass the rope flow through it so that it cannot return to its original position. We continue to exert tension on it, we can use the rope flow to slide it between the thigh and the calf to go to block and secure the other side.

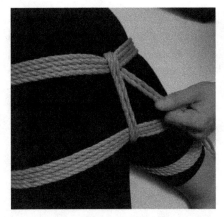

8. From the bottom, we can directly climb the rope flow to the second line of ropes where we will circle this one. This operation will prevent this side from slipping out of the knee.

9. Finally, we can block the rope at the end of the Futomomo by bringing the rope flow to the first line of ropes where we will tie an X knot to block it this way.

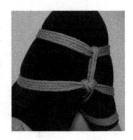

Ebi

This pattern is called Ebi which means shrimp in Japanese. Its main use is to create discomfort by turning a person in on themselves. The goal is not to hurt or injure, but rather to impose a position that allows immobilization. In addition to keeping the arms tied behind the back, the model does not have much room to move. The idea to achieve this is first and foremost to bring your upper body towards the feet. Be careful when imposing this position to respect the model's limits, both psychological ones and those imposed by her body and her flexibility.

There are several levels of difficulty to set it up. We can bet on speed and efficiency or rather on a more complete immobilization bringing at the same time more sensations.

1. To be able to do this position as well as possible, it is best to start by making an upper body harness. Preferably, it should also immobilize the arms behind the back. As we have already seen the TK, you can use this one or one of its variations. You are free to

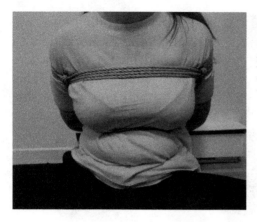

choose another. The model should be in a seated position with the legs crossed with the ankles side by side.

2. We then place a single column tie surrounding the two ankles. In this case, we can make sure that the bight protrudes longer after the knot, since we will be using it later.

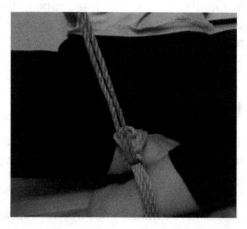

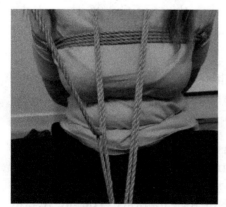

3. With the rope flow we will go to the back of the neck making sure to have the ropes side by side to avoid an overlap which could cause an uncomfortable pressure point. We circulate the rope flow through the bight thus giving us a leverage effect.

4. Slowly, tension is exerted in the rope flow to lower the model's torso while remaining alert for signals indicating discomfort or an inability to continue descending lower. We then turn around to go back to the back of the neck a second time.

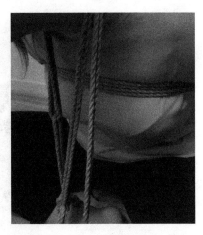

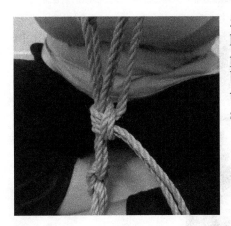

5. We can then exercise a double half hitch to block the rope preventing the model from being able to get up. Although the structure is minimal, it is still sufficient and stable.

By increasing the level of difficulty, we can achieve something generally more comfortable, restrictive, and aesthetic. Thus, we can use two Futomomo for example to immobilize the legs before proceeding to the Ebi position.

1. By keeping the harness at the upper body and adding a Futomomo to each leg, the restriction is increased.

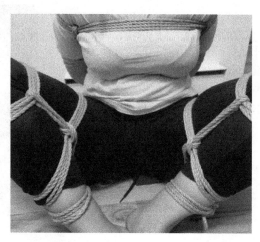

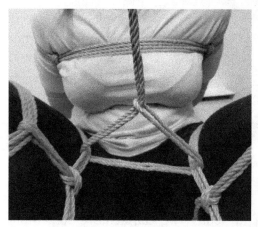

2. We then pass the bight of a new rope through the bottom rope line of each of the two legs, encircling the whole and passing the rope flow through the bight of this same rope.

3. As in the previous example, we are going to skip à back of the neck twice. However, instead of using the bight as a turning point, you can use the bottom of the loop, at the same time increasing the tension between the two legs which will tend to come together.

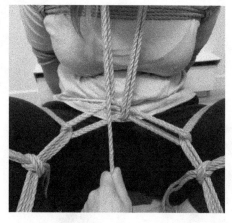

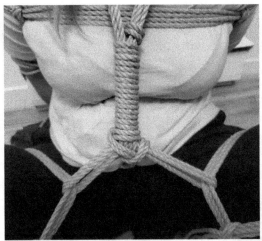

4. To lock this rope, we finish with an X friction knot near the bottom of the loop. If there is any excess left in the rope flow, it can be used to camouflage the ropes going up to the neck by making several turns around them, gradually climbing up to the neck. Be careful not to climb too much. Being close together, the strings will put pressure on the sides of the neck which could cause nerve compression or cut off blood flow to the brain.

The Ebi position may have advantages regarding the restriction but does have some physical dangers that you should be extra careful about. Act with good judgment and remember to avoid unnecessary risks.

Tortoise Shell Tie

This pattern is often used because it embraces the whole body and can thus provide sensations over a large area of the body at the same time. It can be discreet if worn under clothing if it is loose and while wearing a scarf or turtleneck. It is easy to do and can even be done on your own. It is therefore useful if you lack a partner to practice or to tie up when you want to feel the benefits of the rope. These techniques are not highly recommended for making it into suspension unless the structure is reinforced to prevent an accident. Above all, it is about adding aesthetics to the strings. This figure will often be seen in a context to demonstrate bondage as an art highlighting the art and sensations provided by ropes.

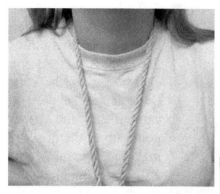

1. We start again with the bight. This time, instead of starting with the doubled rope, we pass the middle of the rope to the back of the neck and where each strand will go to one side of the neck.

2. We will then make a first simple knot towards the base of the neck. It should not be too close to it so as not to cause pressure, but enough so that there is space with the next node.

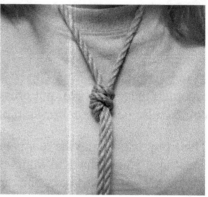

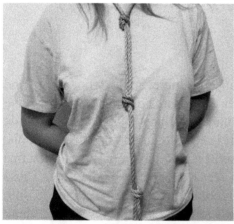

3. The next knot is going to be in the middle of the chest, but for it to end up in this exact location, we will need to place it a few inches below instead. Later, by making diamonds, the knots will naturally come up. It is not impossible that during the first try, the end nodes are not in the place initially desired. From your observations, you can readjust to replace them by adapting them.

4. We are going to form two other nodes while respecting the same distance between each one based on the first two for example.

5. Arriving at the crotch, it is possible to add a step to improve comfort, especially if your model is a woman. This step is therefore optional, and you can skip it completely. Always respecting approximately, the same distance as between the other knots, we will form a chain braiding of three to four loops that will conform to the shape of the crotch. In this case, there will not be a pressure the width of two strands of rope in width, but

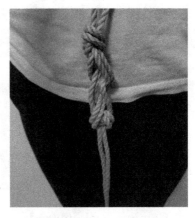

more widely which will distribute the pressure better on the body. The contact will therefore be more pleasant.

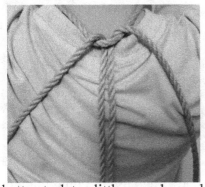

6. The rope flow is circulated to the back of the neck where it is made a U-turn from the bight. From this point on, we will separate the strands of the strings so that each can start from one side of the body. Since the rope is expected to lose length at the front as it goes, we avoid putting any tension in this step. It is even

better to let a little rope hang down. It will always be possible to readjust the lengths later.

7. On each side, run a strand of the rope flow down the side to the front of the body to pass through the first loop between the knot at the neck and the knot at the chest. Each of the strands will turn around one strand of the loop back to the original direction. To prevent the strands from slipping over

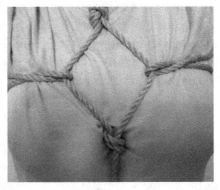

each other, you can do half hitches each time you go through a loop.

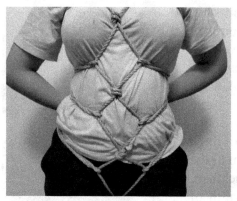

8. In the back, we continue to circulate the strands which return in a straight line, crossing each other and changing sides. From this point, we repeat the previous step until all the loops have been parted forming a series of diamonds.

9. Coming back towards the middle of the back for the last from the last diamond, we will make an X knot in the lower back with the rope running along the spine. Before forming the knot that will permanently maintain the structure, we can make readjustments by exerting tension on the strings to make them more stable

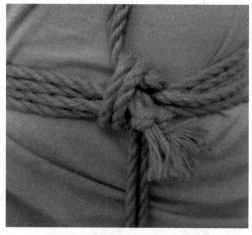

and tauter, but without being too tight. Otherwise, it could quickly become uncomfortable and you should probably detach sooner than expected.

10. If you have rope flow left, you can then wrap it around the vertical rope running down the middle of the back or around the one running horizontally at the lower back. Your strategy depends on how much rope you have left.

The number of diamonds on the front can easily be changed. So, you can add or remove as many as you want. Not putting enough in can give the impression of emptiness and putting in too much will seem overloaded. It is up to you to see the proportions of your body, the length of rope you have and your intentions.

If you plan to wear them in public under your clothes, keep in mind that it may become uncomfortable if you have tied the ropes too tight or if you are sweating. Although it is not always easy to prevent this kind of situation, the ideal is then to walk around with a bag where you can store them after removing them in a more private place, such as a toilet for example.

Dragonfly sleeve

By using this technique, the main goal is to restrict the arms to the sides while being elegant. By attaching this way, the sensations are particularly felt in the arms, but without attaching the rest of the body to the body. It can therefore be used with another upper body harness, except the TK which also requires the arms. In general, the most used harness with this pattern is the dragonfly harness which uses the front of the body to further restrict the arms to the flanks.

Since the arms are strained a lot, the risks associated with compressions should always be kept in mind, whether with the brachial plexus, radial nerve, elbows, or wrists. So, pay attention to the tension you put in the strings as well as the exact places where you place them.

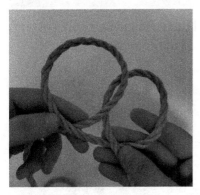

1. From the bight, we first form what is called a Mexican handcuff. We then create two loops from a strand of rope that will be superimposed. One of these two loops which is placed behind the second must be moved to be placed in the front.

2. At the intersection of these two loops are two strands which must each pass through the loop which it does not form. By applying tension to these two strands simultaneously, the center of the handcuff tightens as the curls get larger. It is then possible to adjust the size of these buckles while keeping the center stable so that it can hold the entire handcuff.

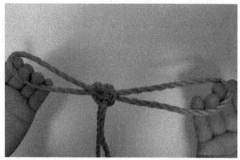

3. With the loops obtained, we will pass the arms through them in the same way as we wear a backpack, by going around the shoulders and passing under the armpits. The center of the handcuff is opposite the spine at the same height as the middle of the shoulders. So, there should be an X shape in the upper back. You can adjust the tension in the ropes from the rope flow. This will then need to be kept constant, both so as not to lose it and to avoid having too many.

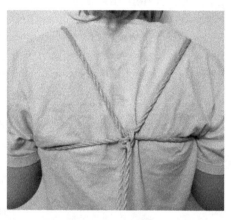

4. A few centimeters lower, we will use the rope flow to make a loop in which we will pass the rope flow. This step can be reminiscent of chain braiding. The difference is that instead of passing the rope flow through this loop again, we will separate the strands to put an arm through each.

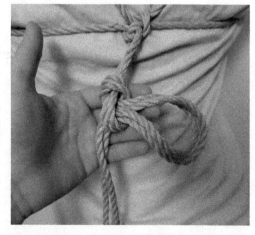

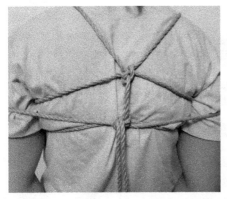

5. The tension in the arms can then be readjusted, still using the rope flow as at the end of step 3.

6. Repeat steps 4 and 5 until you reach the wrists. From this point, one can make a complete readjustment of the tension from the beginning if there would have been a rise or a fall in tension. When everything is satisfied, we can finally block the rope flow by tying an X-shaped knot with the

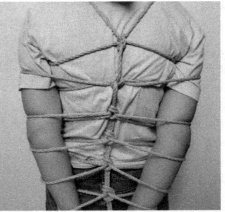

last handcuff, the one at the wrists. The remaining rope flow, if there is any, can be used for something else.

It is up to you how many handcuffs you want to put on. The number can greatly influence depending on the distance you put between each and the size of your model. It is therefore in your judgment to decide what is best for you as well as avoiding the areas of greatest risk.

Armbinder

Slightly resembling the dragonfly sleeve, the armbinder is a technique of restriction of the arms placed in the back. It requires more tension in the ropes and carries a higher risk of compressions. It can be used to require a higher restriction for better control. As the tension is higher, it also causes more sensations, when performed well.

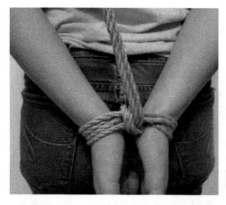

1. Place both arms behind your back, wrists facing each other. The arms do not need to be straight out straight away, they will naturally become so when tension is placed on the ropes. We then form a first anchor point from the wrists with a double column tie. The rope flow must go upwards.

2. We surround an arm for the first time passing over it and which will come back towards the center of the back passing between the side and the arm. We repeat the same action for the other arm. Depending on the number of steps you want to do, you can aim for a height of half or third of the forearm.

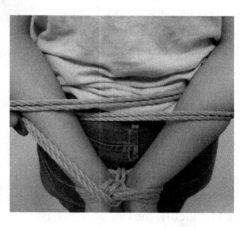

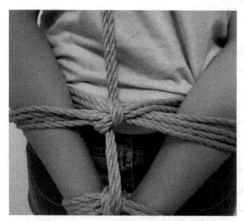

3. We reform this same double loop around the two arms as in the previous step, forming a crossing including all the ropes between the two arms. The rope flow will encircle the rope connecting this line of ropes and the wrists to return to the crossing in the middle of the two arms. Before blocking this level, we want to check that the voltage is regular at each contact with the skin. We will then end up forming an X-shaped friction knot, making sure to collect all the ropes in the process so that there is no slack that can form.

4. From this point on it becomes more important to maintain constant upward tension with the rope flow. As the arms form a V, the loops around them will tend to slide down when there is a lack of upward tension to keep them in place. It can also be quite difficult to replace these once they start to slide. We

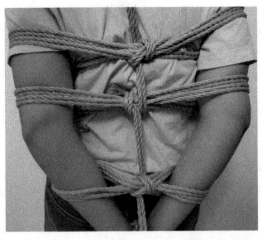

therefore repeat steps 2 and 3 as many times as desired, always making sure to avoid risky points and maintaining constant tension. We stop when the last loop reaches the upper half of the forearms.

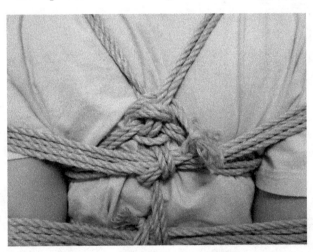

5. Finally, the rope flow must be blocked so that the tension remains constant. Otherwise, at rest, the strings will eventually slip one after the other. To achieve this, we will therefore pass the rope flow over one shoulder to bring it back to the back, passing under the armpit. Then reverse the path, going under the armpit of the second shoulder and coming back over it to come back to the middle of the back. A friction knot 8 is finally formed by encircling the lines joining the top of the shoulders and those of the shoulders.

It is possible to make more than two full turns when circling the arms to provide a larger contact area which will allow better comfort for the model. The number of floors again depends on your intentions and only you can decide what looks best.

To increase the restriction, there is a technique called strict armbinder. As the name suggests, it is more restrictive and therefore also provides more sensations. This technique will not be shown in this guide for safety reasons, as it requires more experience due to the great risk of compressions that accompany it. If the topic is of particular interest to you and you think you are comfortable doing so, you are encouraged to inquire about the topic. Do not attempt to do this if you are not prepared for it.

CONCLUSION

Now you have a huge range of techniques to learn how to handle the strings effectively.

As you continue to practice, you will become even better and can discover methods on your own that can help you improve your creations.

Over time, you will discover the patterns, techniques, and processes that you prefer the most and you will build your own unique style.

Your journey through the Shibari universe is still long and will be filled with pleasure.

Think about safety a lot and have fun, that is most important!